Menopause
Questions and Answers

*The Menopause
Questions and Answers*

SUZANNE BEEDELL

Arlington Books London

THE MENOPAUSE
QUESTIONS AND ANSWERS

first published July 1972 by
Arlington Books (Publishers) Ltd
15/17 King Street, St. James's
London SW1

second impression November 1974
third impression May 1976
fourth impression July 1978
fifth impression February 1980
sixth impression February 1983
seventh impression August 1984

© *Suzanne Beedell 1972*

ISBN 0 85140 203 8

Printed and bound by
The Pitman Press, Bath

To my most understanding husband, Harry

Author's Note

All the quotes in this book, printed in italics, are from statements made by men and women involved in change of life. For obvious reasons all are anonymous.

All medical facts have been checked by a gynaecologist.

My thanks to all those people without whose frank and wholehearted co-operation the book could not have been written.

Contents

Contents—continued

1 Menopause - General Information

The Medical Profession and Change of Life .. Women and Change of Life, and the purpose of this book. .Basic Statistics .. The Basic Endocrinology of Change of Life .. Onset of Menopause .. Abnormalities .. Keeping a Calendar.

Menopause, as most doctors call it, or change of life, as most women call it, is as certain as tomorrow for all women who live through their forties and into their fifties. Yet most young women never even think about it. It is just something which will happen one day, but not yet. Perhaps the fact that it heralds middle age, and ends childbearing, makes the average young woman push the whole subject under the carpet until she reaches forty.

Many of us, as youngsters, lived through the years of a mother's change of life, and watched her experience various strange symptoms which were put down to 'your age, my dear'. If we were deeply worried by it, we may have shut away the thought of our own menopause. Women whose own mothers passed through change without problems often feel that the whole thing is exaggerated, and that they in turn will not be vitally affected. It comes as a bit of a shock if they do develop awkward symptoms in spite of themselves! Equally it comes as a pleasant surprise to some women whose mothers suffered when they themselves sail through it all in unruffled calm.

"I viewed the coming of middle age with some trepidation. My mother's life, and the lives of the family were wrecked with her menopause. Now aged 57, the menopause is well behind me, and apart from a few hot flushes, with never a problem."

What must be stressed here and now is that the one common factor of change of life is that it is different for everyone, and that it is impossible to predict exactly what is going to happen. Although the general symptoms are well known, they come in many permutations.

Menopause comes at what is in any case a difficult time for a woman. Her children are growing up and leaving home, her husband is settled in his job and beginning to think about retirement. Life is settled into a routine. She is facing the fact of declining physical energy as youth passes, (although change of life sometimes increases energy, both mental and physical, for a few years). All the things she has taken for granted, good eyesight and hearing, sound teeth, hair without a strand of grey in it, smooth skin, etc, are failing her. She is being forced to realise that she must now walk when once she could have run. Change of life may seem to set a seal on all these things so that she blames it for everything.

Men, husbands and male doctors, can never directly experience the physical and mental problems of a difficult menopause. It takes a sympathetic and sensitive husband to cope with it, and its repercussions on him and his family. Especially if nobody has ever told them about the physical facts behind change of life, husbands are often totally bewildered by it all, and may become, although loving and sympathetic, absolutely desperate. This book should help such husbands a lot. As for doctors, not emotionally involved with their patients, how much harder it is for them to give a woman the amount of attention which she feels she needs! Some doctors are sympathetic and helpful. Others take the attitude that it is 'just one of those things', and don't offer much more than a few hormones or sedatives in treatment. All doctors will confirm that the permutations of symptoms are enormous and that response to treatment is also extremely variable.

Older doctors will have learnt a lot about change of life from long experience, and from their own wives! But how sympathetic and understanding your doctor may be, will vary. He will know the purely medical treatments, and to which consultants, etc, to pass on extreme cases. He will try to make certain that symptoms are not due to organic troubles other than menopause, which need further attention. He will, for instance, check a palpitating heart for signs of organic heart trouble. But he has other things to do, and however sympathetic he may wish to be, is usually a busy man with a great many patients to attend to; some of whom he knows to be far more seriously ill than women whose symptoms, however distressing, will almost certainly pass in time. He can become impatient of what he may feel to be overdemanding menopausal women on whom he just cannot spend the time that they really need. On the other hand, the 'sympathetic' doctor (and this is always the word which women lucky in their doctors seem to use) probably realises that a word in time saves nine, and will do his best to help a woman, not only directly, but by explaining things to her husband and family as well, as soon as she comes to him for help.

We quote women who have experienced both types of doctor.

"He was generous with his time so that we had a long and intimate talk. I have never been able to unburden myself to anyone as he made me do, and it was such a relief."

"My doctor has no sympathy whatsoever with what he calls my 'neurosis'. He gives me tranquillisers which are useless, and hormones which are even more useless."

"I am indebted to my doctor for the philosophy which sums up my personal findings to date, i.e. immerse yourself in something which interests you and endeavour to set on one side mental and physical inconveniences which may otherwise depress you."

"He is normally most sympathetic, but he merely said that I could have some pills, but wouldn't like their effect."

Comment from a State Registered Nurse, *"I always find that women are so relieved to be talked to about these things instead of merely being handed a pill, which may ease the physical symptoms, but leave the woman in utter bewilderment."*

"Unfortunately doctors have little sympathy or understanding and I think simply feel we are being neurotic."

"I owe a lot to a very sympathetic doctor who gave me mild anti-depressant tablets."

"He gave me some hormone tablets but honestly wasn't in the least interested."

"I would have gone round the bend and collapsed completely without my doctor's help during the recurrent periods of depression and nervous tension during the past 5 years."

"I was lucky with my doctor."

"Somehow I am left with the feeling (and other women agree with me) that despite all that is said, doctors aren't really interested in helping women through this difficult time."

These quotes speak worlds on both sides, and of course one is more likely to hear from women who have not got the help they wanted from their doctors, than from those whose doctors have been helpful and successful.

Our theme is that somehow the problems must be brought out into daylight and women given every chance to air and share their feelings, and that doctors, husbands, families and friends who shut a woman up, or make her feel that she is being foolish, just make matters worse, not only for the patient, but for themselves in the long run. This book is an attempt to air the commonest problems through the words of women themselves. We believe that to know that the problems exist and are recognised is more than half the battle. The rest is up to medical research, particularly in endocrinology; to the social and welfare services, and most certainly to all of us personally involved.

BASIC FACTS

There are those who hate to hear menopause referred to as 'change of life' because they believe that this predisposes women to expect a total change in their lives, which in fact is not going to happen. This belief makes two wrong assumptions. First, that women must think that 'change' always means 'change for the worse' and not 'change for the better'. It can and often does mean 'change for the better'. Secondly, that no change occurs, when everyone knows that there is a change, even if it is only that one has no more periods and no more children. The medical term 'menopause' can be equally misleading for those who don't know its origin. The woman who does not know that monthly periods are called 'menses' or 'menstruation' won't realise that menopause is a word from the same latin root, meaning 'the end of menstruation' and could even translate it as being something to do with pausing as far as men are concerned!! Perhaps that sounds ridiculous, but it is just as logical as the objection to the term 'change of life'. One other term frequently used is 'climacteric' meaning 'a critical point of life'. Physiologically it means 'a period of decrease in reproductive capacity in men and women, culminating in women in the menopause'. It isn't really quite the right word, especially as some people automatically feel that a climax is a high point from which one can go nowhere but down. So it comes back to 'change of life' which is the most generally accepted term, the one which ordinary men and women use. Menopause is a nice short easy word to use, and so in this book, the two terms are interchangable.

Research into menopause has been patchy, and not on anything like the scale that is devoted to many other serious medical and social problems. Change of life is not a killer disease, to which most research must be devoted. Discoveries of treatments for menopausal symptoms often do come as by-products of research into other things.

STATISTICS

15% of women pass right through change of life with no physical or mental difficulties at all.

85% have symptoms varying from slight to very severe.

At any given time, 1 in 8 women in this country are menopausal.

Treatments, both physical and mental are successful in some cases and not in others.

Whatever symptoms one has are never unique. Millions of other women have them as well. For many women menopause is a time when they get a new lease of life, a resurgence of creative activity; an enormous sense of freedom from the responsibilities of childbearing, and a chance to be very useful citizens in other respects.

It cannot be stressed too strongly that anyone experiencing any symptoms should seek medical help, for there is in fact much that can be done in most cases; and it is vital that checks are made to ensure a clean bill of health in other respects.

PHYSICAL FACTS OF CHANGE OF LIFE.

The female reproductive system is controlled from birth to death by the endocrine glands which manufacture and secrete hormones; chemicals which exercise control over all our bodily functions. The efficiency, productivity and output of these glands are responsible, directly or indirectly for controlling us astronomically complex creatures. In other words, they make us tick! Research is going on continuously, all over the world, into the endocrines and their hormones. Much is still not known, much is known but not completely understood. As far as women and menopause is concerned, the ideal, which no doubt medical science will one day achieve, would be to assess exactly the endocrine processes and balances of each individual and to be able to correct imbalances so that everything could proceed smoothly and without trouble.

From puberty, when the monthly periods (menstruation) begin, the body's hormones stimulate the ovaries to release an egg cell every month. This egg travels through the fallopian tubes to the womb, which has at the same time been hormonally stimulated to thicken its lining. Should the egg be fertilised by meeting a male sperm, this lining will receive the egg and begin the processes of pregnancy. If no fertilisation occurs, the thickened lining disintegrates, and there is a loss of blood which removes it and the unfertilised egg, as a monthly period. The hormone which stimulates all this is largely oestrogen, manufactured in the ovarian glands themselves, but governed in turn by hormones from the thyroid gland (situated in the neck) and by the master gland, which is the pituitary gland in the base of the skull. The ovarian glands also create other substances which in turn have a controlling effect upon the oestrogen. This simple summary is enough to show how all the processes are very complicated and interlocked.

As the supply of eggs in the ovaries runs out (every woman is born with the eggs which she will shed during life, and no more are created during her life) and nature decides that a woman is approaching the age when she is unsuitable for childbearing, the contribution of oestrogen from the ovaries diminishes and the whole process slows down. Eventually no more eggs are released, so no more thickened womb lining builds up, and menstruation ceases. But because oestrogen and all the hormones have other effects on the body, unless the oestrogen is replaced in some way, other physical and mental troubles may result. Normally the body re-adjusts itself. The suprarenal glands also produce some oestrogen and they take over some of the work of the ovaries in this respect, and if the take-over goes smoothly, no difficult symptoms will occur. In the long run, the endocrine system does adjust itself, and although ageing continues, as the hormone output is reduced, one can remain perfectly healthy and balanced physically for the rest of life. If the changing hormone pattern doesn't go smoothly, then symptoms occur, and at present doctors prescribe hormones either extracted from glands, or manufactured synthetically in laboratories to try to help out the glands, while nature takes its course.

On the face of it, this would seem to be a fine and easily applied solution; but as we have said above the problem is to assess exactly which hormone, and how much of it a woman needs. At present this seems to be a bit of a hit or miss process. For some women hormone pills or injections do reduce such symptoms as hot flushes, and have a definite rejuvenating effect upon skin, hair, etc, without unpleasant side effects. In others they may occasionally produce unwanted pigmentation, and often restart periods, which, although no egg is present, may make it hard for a woman to decide whether or not she should continue with contraception. In any case the continuance of periods is nothing but an unmitigated nuisance. There is a school of thought in America which recommends feeding women oestrogen pills regularly before, during and after menopause, claiming that this minimises symptoms, slows down the obvious side effects of ageing, and generally gives women a new lease of life. The exponents of this have by no means proved their case, and do not go out of their way to report their failures. While not wishing to condemn prolonged oestrogen treatments out of hand, we must stress that they are NOT the final answer.

"I started having flushes and periods stopped. I had some pills, and found them effective, but they restarted periods."

"The hormone pills seemed to cause a complete change of personality, and I soon felt so unbalanced and so unsure of myself that I became really desperate."

"I was having flushes every 30 minutes every day. My doctor prescribed hormone pills which were a great help. The flushes only returned for 2 or 3 days every fourth week when I had to leave off the pills. I have moved, and my new doctor decided I must not have any more pills, so now I am having 15 or 16 hot flushes per day."

What works for some, doesn't work for others. There is no rule of thumb, no certainty, except that the symptoms will eventually pass, and that in themselves they are not killers.

Our human problem is how to deal with them both medically and in terms of emotions and feelings until the body sorts itself out.

ONSET OF MENOPAUSE.

There is absolutely no telling when a woman will start or finish menopause.

"My G.P. assured me that a lot of women were starting the menopause later—the whole thing being bound up with our youthful way of life nowadays, and our mental outlook!"

It is unusual but not unknown for it to begin in the late thirties; but it starts more often in the middle and late forties, and can continue well into the middle and late fifties. It can even delay its onset until the middle fifties. *"I have been absolutely regular at 27 days ever since I was 11½. I am now 54 and missed one month 8 months ago—and have missed 4 months this summer."*

VARIOUS WAYS IN WHICH MENSTRUATION CEASES

1. Menstruation just ceases abruptly and no further periods or bleeding follow.
2. The menstrual flow gradually lessens and tails right off till it ceases entirely, but there is no irregularity of periods.
3. Normal periods occur, but occasionally one is missed until they cease altogether.
4. Periods gradually lessen and at the same time are occasionally missed completely.
5. Normal periods are followed by a few months of no periods, and then more normal periods, and then another gap until the final gap lengthens into a complete cessation.
6. The length of the cycle will alter and the regular

twenty-eight day occurence will become more frequent, say twenty-five days or even a fortnight late.

ABNORMALITIES.

If any woman suffers bleeding which for her is unusual, she should consult a doctor, for there are various conditions which can cause this and which can be put right. Many women fear cancer at menopause and worry themselves desperately about it, usually unnecessarily. Medical and surgical examination and the regular taking of cervical smears by your doctor can set your mind at rest, or ensure that if there is any trouble it can be dealt with swiftly and effectively.

Conditions which should be investigated
1. Prolonged bleeding, lasting longer than a week.
2. Excessive flooding with or without heavy clots.
3. Irregular bleeding between periods.
4. Bleeding on straining or on intercourse.
5. Any kind of spotting or discharge.

It is important not to wait and see if the condition clears up by itself, but to pay a visit to your doctor straight away. He would far rather deal with these symptoms at their onset than when they have worsened and become acute. From your point of view it is foolishness to feel that you should not worry your doctor over something which may be trivial and to continue to worry yourself into a state, probably needlessly. So if you are worried, go to the doctor.

2 Physical Problems

Flushes and Sweats . . Heart Sensations . .
Tingling . . Giddiness . . Headaches . . Rheumatic Pains . . Obesity . . Indigestion . . Flatulence . . Facial Hair . . Skin Irritations . . Pigmentation . . Vaginal Irritation . . Fatigue . .
Malaise.

The physical symptoms of change of life take many
forms and occur by themselves or in combinations. Many
women have no symptoms at all; others may have some of
the symptoms for reasons other than change of life. For
instance, someone who suffers from chronic arthritis
cannot blame it on change when it continues through that
time, although the sudden onset of arthritis during
menopause may be related to it.

HOT FLUSHES WHY DO THEY HAPPEN?

Hot flushes are the commonest of menopausal symptoms and about 60% of women have them. Almost every
woman who has other symptoms has hot flushes to
contend with as well, yet for many they are the only
symptom. They are probably due to the reduced amounts
of oestrogen failing to counterbalance certain stimuli from
the pituitary gland. Consequently one feels a flush of
warmth followed by sweating. Now this can be quite
slight, just like a deep blush, which is all you see in the

mirror. Not unnaturally women who have a lot of hot flushes feel that other people notice them and are sometimes acutely embarrassed because of associations with sexual matters. In any case the flush and the consequent sweating are unpleasant even though they are usually not half so noticeable to others as the sufferer feels them to be. The occasional flush isn't too bad, but women who have to put up with a great many, perhaps for years on end, do get thoroughly demoralised and upset.

WHEN DO THEY HAPPEN?

Hot flushes can happen at any time of life if oestrogen balance is disturbed, and some middle-aged men get them too. They may happen before menopause really begins yet not be present during the years of change. They may reappear or start after menopause has finished, or persist right through change. Some women suffer just a few, others have a great many; and know by a feeling of tension just when a flush is imminent. The main thing to remember is that they are not in the least dangerous, and that in the enormous majority of cases will disappear in due course.

HOW FREQUENT WILL THEY BE?

One woman of 58 reports hot flushes for 8 years which make her very depressed, occuring as often as a dozen times a day and throughout the night. *"Often I find myself bursting into a profuse sweat in the middle of a conversation with a stranger and am desperate with misery and embarrassment."* She has only very slight problems otherwise, but her doctor has been unable to help her and two specialists were *"both very kind, but neither of them was able to give me any practical help."*

Another woman reports having flushes when periods stopped, but on taking oestrogen tablets, although the flushes stopped, periods restarted, *"Since then I have continued with flushes but have learned to live with them as they are merely annoying."* She is 59.

A woman whose flushes became unbearable, and was given hormones, complained of a change of personality and stopped taking the hormones. *"Then the physical symptoms took over again and the exhaustion of violent flushing, the face so wet that glasses will not stay in place, the hair stuck to the scalp, stockings to the legs."*

On the other side of the record, we know of many women who had had no flushes at all, and wonder what all the fuss is about. *"Hot flushes as such, I have never had."* Others have flushes but find that they are adequately controlled by hormone tablets prescribed by the doctor without adverse side effects. One woman states that *"herb tablets"* control her flushes.

NIGHT SWEATS

Many women have hot flushes and sweats at night which keep them awake, with consequent tiredness and depression due to loss of sleep. One woman actually says that her night-time flushes keep her warm in bed, so she doesn't mind a bit, which is perhaps a good way of minimising the problem.

"I would wake at night and feel overfull, and a kind of discomfort which caused me to be hot, and sweat, would last moments, and then pass. I would sleep again and try to forget, but its recurrence was frequent, and I wondered rather miserably whether this heralded something more dire." This quote is extremely descriptive of what happens and of how it starts a sequence of worry.

COLD FLUSHES

These take the form of a cold sweat, not preceeded by hot feelings and blushing, and are, although unpleasant for the sufferer, not noticeable to others and therefore less embarrassing.

MEDICAL TREATMENT OF FLUSHES

Medical treatments will consist of oestrogen tablets or injections, or of general sedatives. Your doctor should be able to sort out with you which treatment works best. The woman who has always tended to sweat when she is nervous, or shy, or tense, will probably respond to mild sedatives as well as she will to hormones.

HOW ONE CAN UNDERSTAND AND COPE WITH FLUSHES

These extremely unpleasant and embarrassing happenings are not dangerous. They can usually, though not always, be controlled medically. And perhaps most important of all, can loom far less large if accepted as a matter of course, without worry. If they are noticeable to others, try hard to train yourself into a 'couldn't care less if they do notice' attitude. Plenty of baths talcum powder and deodorants, containing anti-perspirants, go a long way to counteract the unhygienic effects of constant sweating. Also wear cotton nightdresses and underwear, not nylon, as cotton is more absorbent.

Remember all the time that flushes will eventually lessen and pass away. The trouble is that if they go on for years, it is desperately hard to keep one's spirits up endlessly, just as it is desperately hard for the teenager with bad acne to wait until the condition dies away as the hormones balance out.

NERVOUS DISORDERS OF THE HEART, PALLOR, FAINTNESS, NUMBNESS, TINGLING SENSATIONS, PALPITATIONS, ETC.

"Dreadful feelings of faintness and weakness would sweep over me as if at any moment my knees would give way." This kind of remark is common from menopausal women, and there are those who are quite certain that they are suffering from some kind of heart disease and are about to drop down dead at any moment. There may be attacks of palpitation, or the heart races for a while. The heart may give a kind of hiccup. These symptoms aren't usually so noticeable when one is active, but come when resting or just before sleep.

WHY THEY OCCUR

These symptoms are NOT those of heart disease and are seldom associated with it. They are in fact common in anyone under nervous strain, and particularly during change of life. It is just a fact, but because we all know that our hearts have got to keep going, these sensations are horrible and rather frightening.

TREATMENT

Your doctor will check your heart and blood pressure and reassure you about the causes of the symptoms, and will probably prescribe a sedative. Of course there just might be something really wrong, and such a check will enable him to treat it, but it really is more than likely that there is absolutely nothing wrong, nothing to fear. When the symptoms occur, if you are already resting, continue to do so, and if not resting, sit down for a bit, take it easy, but don't worry. Try not to listen to your own heart beat, or the nervous tension will make it worse.

OTHER CONDITIONS
WHY THEY OCCUR

"Briefly, my physical symptoms have been as follows: palpitations, vertigo and fainting, middle ear trouble, tingling, breathlessness and sore chest muscles."

The lesser symptoms of fidgetyness, tingling in the extremities, are also partly nervous in origin and due to oestrogen imbalance. *"Sudden attack of the fidgets, tingling and aching in feet, hands and limbs, and severe cramp in feet, calves and thighs at night."* These plague menopausal women and cause loss of sleep and tiredness and all the things that go with it, including a dread of the night time and going to sleep for fear of being woken by the symptoms.

WHEN THEY OCCUR

All these symptoms will pass in due course as the hormones balance themselves, and will probably only occur during the menopausal years, not before. And never to anything like the extent that hot flushes may do.

TREATMENT

Your doctor may prescribe hormone treatment, sedatives or tranquillisers, and again worry only makes things worse.

GIDDINESS

Giddiness and vertigo are experienced by 40% of women during change of life, and usually only mildly. If you normally suffer from vertigo (just can't stand heights) you will know the feeling. To be on top of a high building or a cliff or even something harmless like a flight of open steps, induces a terrifying feeling of loss of balance, sometimes so acute that you feel sick or fall down or even faint.

WHY?

This is caused by disturbance of the human balance

mechanism in the inner ear, and slight alteration of circulation in the area will start it off, and this can happen during menopause.

"I also experience feelings of giddiness. (I do not suffer from hypertension)."

Those normally liable to attacks of vertigo may find they become worse during menopause. *"I never liked heights very much, but I was taken by surprise when I first suffered a very severe attack of vertigo when sightseeing on Westminster Cathedral tower, and subsequently on other high places. This had not happened before change of life, and not yet having passed through the state, I do not know when the present irrational terror of heights and feelings of giddiness will pass. I do know that if, when they happen, I sit tight, and rest awhile, the physical and mental symptoms disappear after about 10 minutes. I have photos taken looking vertically down on Cologne from the top of the cathedral to prove it. Ten minutes before taking them, I could not stand up, let alone walk up the last flight of steps."*

TREATMENT

Ask your doctor to check if you suffer these symptoms, for giddiness can be caused by ear trouble or by high blood pressure. If he can rule out these causes he will probably prescribe tablets which do help a lot with this problem.

HEADACHES

Headaches are very common menopausal symptoms,

especially in those already prone to them. *"I'm conscious all the time of a vague headache."* is the cry of so many menopausal women.

They may be caused by any number of things.

1. By the mid-forties, the eyes are probably getting a bit weak and could be causing trouble.

2. Usually headaches spring from tiredness, strain, anxiety and nervous tension, and all these things will be exaggerated during change of life.

3. Those who have always suffered from migraine may find that it worsens during change of life, and then disappears altogether. It is a comfort to women who have suffered from migraine most of their young lives to know that change of life will bring them relief from it in the long run. Other women experience migraine occasionally ONLY during change of life. Only she who has had migraine headaches really knows just how frightful they are.

"The next thing was headaches always on the same side. A feeling as though something was boring through my right eye. I get them every three weeks and they last 24 hours, and I feel sick."

TREATMENT

Consult your doctor and describe the type of headache you have been getting, and he will prescribe accordingly. Headaches can be dealt with very successfully, although it may not be possible for your doctor to prevent the onset of bad migraine, he will be able to alleviate it when it happens.

Do not take excessive or regular daily doses of pain killers—asprins, codein compounds, phenacatin, bought over a chemist's counter, without consulting your doctor.

Avoid strain, worry and overtiredness and over-excitement, especially when you feel a headache coming on. Take what painkillers have been prescribed for you, to prevent a slight headache developing into a snorter.

RHEUMATIC PAINS AND ARTHRITIS

The term 'rheumatic' covers a multitude of aches and pains, including fibrositis, and odd aches in the limbs. These may be caused by obesity or thyroid deficiency. Undoubtedly some women do become arthritic during menopause, but this may be due to other organic causes, and natural ageing.

Quite apart from the unpleasantness of pain itself, these rheumatic pains, especially for someone who has never suffered them before, are very depressing, as they seem to be such a sign of approaching old age.

"At the same time as all this (menopause) started, I began with arthritis, particularly in my hands, but am pleased to say since taking cider vinegar and honey every day, the arthritis is under control."

TREATMENT

Hormone and asprin can have dramatic effects on these conditions and here the doctor should really be able to help, but rheumatic conditions which are truly due to menopause will clear up to a great extent as the hormones balance out and such as do persist into later life, are probably not menopausal in origin. Take pain killers only as prescribed by your doctor.

OBESITY

At least 40% of women put on weight and inches during change of life, and it is a fact that married women put on more weight than single women.

WHY?

There are various causes of obesity.

1. Sheer overeating. Often nervous in origin. The first reaction of some women when worried, is to go and eat something, just as others reach for the nearest cigarette.

2. Energy is running out a bit by middle forties, and some women do feel very tired during menopause, so they take much less exercise. Sometimes the departure of children and lessening of family responsibilities and work encourage her to take it easy and just get plain lazy!

3. Thyroid deficiency at menopause can cause obesity.

4. Fluid retention in the body cells may increase at change of life. *"My ankles and feet became very swollen and hardly ever went back into shape."*

"I reckon that gaining weight is connected with the menopause and is caused by retention of liquid in the tissues. I am attempting to change my eating habits to counteract this and have started to do exercises; and results are encouraging."

TREATMENT

Obesity, generally speaking, is an extremely difficult problem for men and women of all ages, and not enough is known about it for treatment to be successful in every case.

Carefully controlled diet, low on starch and sugar, and calories, will help many to reduce weight, but leave others quite unreduced. These need special diets under medical supervision.

Getting rid of fluids in Turkish baths, or by taking diuretic pills which cause much urine to be passed, only helps obesity temporarily, and such fluid is almost immediately replaced by the next few cups of tea or whatever. However treatment with diuretic pills may be essential in severe cases of oedema.

It is obviously important therefore, that your doctor makes a great effort to find out from what kind of obesity you are suffering, and to prescribe a special diet. It is equally important, if fluid retention and oedema are the problems, that fluid intake is limited to 2 pints a day. The body cannot retain fluid without salt to help it, so cut the salt and less fluid is retained. Salt substitutes can be bought but are not really very palatable, and it is not too hard to learn to do without, or to use other non-salty flavourings.

Obesity due to thyroid deficiency can be corrected by treatment with thyroid hormones.

CONCLUSION

Because obesity in itself can lead to so many other troubles as it puts a strain on the heart and circulation, it really is important to try to control it. Yet there are those who seem to be able to carry their weight and are healthier fat than when under the constant mental and physical strain of diet routines. Make up your own mind with the help of your doctor and try to find a compromise between excessive weight and excessive dieting. Perhaps the worst part of it for women is that clothes won't fit and girdles and bras become tight and uncomfortable and one interprets this as another sign of approaching old age. The constant struggle to become sylph-like again puts a big strain on the nerves. Many of the best dressed and most elegant women are not young and sylph-like at all, they have just come to terms with the figure changes of their middle years!

Those women who actually lose weight during menopause usually do so because worry and the discomfort of other symptoms just puts them off food. Cooking smells disgust them as they do pregnant women, and they simply eat less and lose weight, just as if they were deliberately dieting. *"I have actually lost two stone, which is probably due to the fact that I just don't fancy food because of internal upsets."* The weight loss will probably do nothing but good, unless it becomes extreme; but take care to eat a balanced diet, if a limited one, and not to live on snacks and odds and ends.

DIGESTIVE TROUBLES, FLATULENCE, DISTENTION, CONSTIPATION.

The woman who has never suffered from chronic indigestion, stomach ulcers, flatulence, constipation, etc, but who does so during change of life may be developing organic trouble of some kind. Consult your doctor if these symptoms occur—just to make certain that there is nothing really wrong. Worry about other symptoms can cause digestive upsets; and throughout life, worry or strain of any kind can lead to nervous gastritis, or even to stomach ulcers.

"I constantly know a dull sick feeling, and a great deal of flatulence, which causes great distress."

"I suffer dreadfully from flatulence. I can pass wind neither up nor down and it causes considerable distention, and it is as if the wind is causing pressure on other parts internally and even gives me a weak feeling in the legs."

"I suffer from perpetual stomach upsets with a dull feeling of sickness, and being unable to face food. I get days when my bowels work overtime."

These are typical quotes, and often the symptoms complained of are not unlike those of pregnancy. Slight indigestion and liverishness, almost like a mild hangover!

WHY?

Hormone imbalance may be affecting the digestive processes directly, but it is far more likely to be worry, combined with less exercise, and possibly unbalanced diet, which is causing the trouble. Women who live alone sometimes get less and less interested in feeding themselves and live on snacks, or on the other hand, overeat compulsively as a kind of reaction against worry and loneliness. Even women with families, once their children depart and their husbands need less food as they too become less athletic and active, don't bother to cook such regular or such balanced meals. Too many cups of tea or coffee, more alcohol, heavier smoking, may well upset the digestion. Strictly speaking, therefore, one can't blame it all on menopause.

TREATMENT

Careful diet, if necessary as suggested by your doctor, and avoidance of food and drink which you know to be indigestable for you personally, and medical treatment as prescribed, will do a very great deal to help. Either in the form of medicine to aid digestion, or sedatives or tranquillisers to stop you worrying.

DON'T take regular doses of tablets or powders bought over the counter of a chemists or grocers without prescription, especially those containing asprin, phenacetin, or codein compounds. Taken occasionally these products relieve pain and some other symptoms, but taken regularly and excessively they can cause serious digestive upsets including interior bleeding. They should not be taken in an attempt to *cure* indigestion. As a golden rule, never take regular or excessive doses of any drug without a doctor's prescription.

FACIAL HAIR

Occasionally, again due to hormone changes, facial hair increases during change of life, single coarse hairs grow, or fine downy hair increases. Most women find this embarrassing and ugly. *"I was conscious of brown spots on my face, hairs appearing on my lip and chin, sagging muscles and wrinkles. I seemed to age ten years in a few months."*

"I am continually saddened by people who too easily describe someone as 'a bit long in the tooth' or 'grey-haired and with a moustache to match', and I always wonder why the observer doesn't recognise 'but for the grace of God, there go I'."

TREATMENT

Pluck out single hairs with tweezers, and remove the downy hair with depilatory wax. Really troublesome single hairs can be removed permanently by electrolysis. None of these treatments stimulate the growth of hair as is commonly believed, and do not create a 'stubble'. Even the occasional shave in bad cases does not make the growth worse. If this were so, then men, who shave daily, would end up with the most fantastic growth rate of facial hair, and this of course doesn't happen.

SKIN IRRITATIONS

All kinds of skin disorders arise during menopause, from psoriasis to wrinkles. *"All of a sudden, and it seemed overnight, my skin was changing. I noticed my forearms getting crinkled instead of smooth, and my neck was changing in the same way. Under my eyes I was aware of a new person emerging."*

"I have just had a month's treatment at a skin hospital which has cured the psoriasis for the time being anyway."

"My troubles began when I was 49 with nettlerash."

Patches of irritation can occur anywhere, but particularly around the genitals.

WHY?

Lack of oestrogen and hormone imbalance is probably the cause, because anxiety states can lead to skin troubles, and oestrogen lack can lead to anxiety states. This is yet another indication of the interlocking of physical and mental symptoms which crop up all the time.

TREATMENT

Injections of hormones, hormone tablets, or even local treatment with hormone creams may help a lot. Don't scratch itchy places. Feed your face with hormone skin creams as recommended by cosmetic manufacturers, according to your choice. Even those who have never bothered to take much care of their skin will benefit from continual skin care from the forties on.

PIGMENTATION

Skin colour, whether you are fair skinned, olive skinned, brown skinned, or black, depends on pigmentation. In some women pigmentation collects in small patches or freckles, thoughout life, and at change of life these freckles may become marked. Patches of pigmentation may occur spontaneously, and some women feel them to be very unsightly. There isn't much to be done about this problem, and it is rarely unsightly at all. In fact some people find freckles extremely attractive. Occasionally extra pigmentation may occur when taking hormone treatments, and should this happen to you, report it to your doctor. There is nothing dangerous about it, but he will probably take you off the hormone to stop the freckles getting worse.

VAGINAL IRRITATION AND CYSTITIS

An extreme case reports considerable vaginal discomfort. *"One of the worst things I endure is a kind of muscular spasm and contractions in the vagina itself. Sometimes I feel I am going to turn inside out! This comes at recurring intervals. Externally I am acutely conscious of a feeling of pins and needles all over the whole area, and at times this even extends to the anus. Often too there is an acute burning sensation and flickering of nerves."*

"I find I get days when my bladder seems irritated and I get a feeling like an electric current running through the passage when I pass water, and I am spending a penny every few minutes."

It has been recognised that some forms of cystitis are nervous in origin, and many non-menopausal women suffer this disability. Such women develop these symptoms, and even more acute ones when they are worried or upset. Consult your doctor.

FATIGUE AND GENERAL MALAISE

Many women complain of continual weariness during change of life. *"I feel so tired quite suddenly, that when I sat down I used to think that if the house were on fire, I wouldn't have the energy to get up."*

WHY?

Sometimes this is due to a state of permanent thyroid deficiency especially among women who have worked hard physically for years. They have slowed down mentally and physically and everything has genuinely become too much for them. So much so that they accept the state of affairs and don't even try to get family or friends to help them out physically with work, or their doctors to prescribe treatment.

Tiredness is also linked with all kinds of mental anxiety and with insomnia or interrupted sleep caused by hot flushes, and aches and pains. *"I have a daily rest in the afternoon so that I could present my best side to the family in the evening."*

TREATMENT

It is usual that medical treatment for some other menopausal condition will at the same time help the patient to feel less tired, because the causes of tiredness are so widespread. Sleep as long as possible, and if necessary rest occasionally during the day. Recourse to 'pick me ups' isn't the answer, and constant cups of tea, coffee, or alcoholic drinks produce other problems and won't do anything but make one feel a little better for a very little while.

MALAISE

Perhaps not so marked or identifiable as fatigue, yet probably the most common symptom of all, especially in women who are not suffering severe symptoms, is what can only be described as malaise. "Uneasiness", doesn't translate the word, nothing does, but those who suffer will know. It's just a general feeling of not being 100%. Perhaps very slightly sick, very slightly headachy, very slightly liverish. Some women have had the same feeling during pregnancy, not amounting to real sickness, but none the less enough to make them very definitely off colour. A bit like a slight hangover! These feelings are probably due to slight hormone imbalance, and not to the onset of some dire disease, and usually disappear at least temporarily on involvment in some activity, mental or physical. The trouble is that to make the effort to get involved is difficult when you aren't feeling up to it in the first place, even though you know that you'll feel better if you do. It's a vicious circle!

3 Mental Problems

Premenstrual Tension . . Anxiety . . Tear-
fulness . . Irrational Fears . . Truculence
. . Inadequacy and Depression . .
Thoughts of Death . . How to Cope.

PREMENSTRUAL TENSION

Every woman knows that each month during her adult
life, as her periods approach and recede, she changes. For a
few days before a period she suffers from tender breasts,
and perhaps from stomach distention or slight oedema.
She may also get very nervy and irritable. If she has been
lucky enough to have had the state explained to her, she
will know that the physical changes are due to hormone
changes before the period begins, and that the premenstrual tension and irritability, also have the same
physical basis. The sufferer from premenstrual tension,
who knows it, finds it much easier to laugh off or apologise
for an outburst of temper, because she and her family
know why it happened, or at any rate why it was probably
exaggerated out of all proportion to its cause.

Women know that a sudden shock, or even a physical
illness such as a feverish cold may bring on a period, or
perhaps prevent one from appearing, and if they have
asked their doctors about it, understand that this too is
due to hormone imbalance caused by shock or anxiety. So

it all works both ways, normal physical changes produce hormone changes which produce physical and mental symptoms. You can only win, really, by knowing what is happening and not being frightened by it. Throughout adult life until menopause, most women cheerfully accept these facts. Yet when change of life starts off exactly the same kinds of sequence of hormone imbalance and anxieties, all kinds of nervous states of mind follow, as well as the physical symptoms. It is most unfair for people to say 'well, it's just nerves'. Of course it is just nerves, but nerves brought on by hormone imbalance. At the same time, while it is equally unfair to say 'pull yourself together, you'll be better if you get a grip on yourself' when someone finds it almost impossible to do this, the state of mind of the sufferer does have an enormous bearing on how well or how badly she copes with her troubles.

ANXIETIES

The first and most important thing to understand is that these many menopausal symptoms have their origin in hormone imbalance in turn exaggerated by anxieties. *"The aspect of the condition that disturbs me more than the strange physical discomforts has been the realisation that the erratic supply or lack of it, of different hormones alters one's entire personality. One has no free will any more."* Having recognised the roots of her problems, this woman is still upset and fighting against them, rather than accepting them. *"Vanished is what one fondly 'thought'*

*was one's normal self, and instead a lump of depressed
dough, completely lacking in enthusiasm and self confidence, has to plod inefficiently through the work of the
following days, with no hope of the black clouds lifting.
This has led me to the conclusion that free will is a
myth—we are indeed puppets on strings pulled by the
changing glandular balance over which we have no
conscious control."*

This statement from one who has thought a lot about
herself is very extreme, and she has a lot more to say in the
same vein. It is self pity, yet she knows it is self pity and
finds it impossible to pull out. Yet undoubtedly as her
hormones balance themselves or if she gets effective
medical treatment, she will pull out of this slough of
despond, and one day will wonder what it was all about.
Meanwhile, although she understands her condition, she is
still suffering.

Such books as have been written on the subject, such
treatment as doctors or psychologists can offer, tend to be
hopefully reassuring and palliative, but do not face up to
the fact that although treatments, doses of hormones,
sympathetic and reassuring words may help some, they do
not help all women, and that for the ones who are not so
helped, it is no good sweeping things under the carpet. It
all has to be aired and faced up to and understood by
everyone concerned, the woman, her family and friends,
and her doctor.

Both sides of the problem must be put. *"At 51, with*

two grown up sons, a widow for the last six years forced to earn my own living, I am still wondering what the menopause is all about. My lifelong hay fever has become rare. Premenstrual tension is far less marked, even breast soreness is no longer apparent. My figure even without dieting, has not altered."

"I am now over sixty, married with three children, enjoy a normal sex life, have had no headaches, hot flushes, etc, my periods have faded out, and I have taken up writing most successfully."

TEARFULNESS

There are all kinds of emotional upsets. Some women find that they weep easily and for no reason, although this can let off steam a bit. *"I used to consider myself phlegmatic. I have heard myself described as serene, but now find I tend to be emotional and find myself weeping over books, plays, films; and am easily moved to tears. Quite embarrassing this, at times."*

"I was in a complete panic, lost all sense of proportion and collapsed in fits of tears and shivering if the slightest thing went wrong; I also felt loads of guilt for little peccadilloes in my past life, and expected every day to bring dire punishment."

IRRATIONAL FEARS

Irrational fears are a great problem. Those who suffer them seem to know perfectly well that they are being irrational, but cannot control them. One woman reports having to leave various jobs, being unable to use public transport, or to enter heated shops, libraries and offices because, *"most of all I cannot bear the fluorescent lighting which all offices seem to have, not to mention the terrible heat everywhere."*

Another, ten years after her periods ceased has, *"a terrible fear of going to the dentist, optician, etc, which is very frightening because I am now sixty-two and must have my eyes and teeth attended to from time to time. I have cancelled appointments because this horrible fear possessed my whole mind and body—and it is fear! I am a religious woman and cannot even go to church, unless I sit very near the door!"* These fears take all kinds of shapes and forms, but seem to be mainly claustrophobic, (an exaggerated fear of being shut in anywhere) or a deep resentment against getting old, expressed in the case above as a fear of being told that teeth or sight are getting very bad. Other women, even those who have lived a life of social and public work, develop a fear of people, and cannot face them any longer.

"I wanted to avoid people and just keep in my own four walls, yet I used to be a cinema/bingo manageress. I do try desperately to make an effort to shake myself out of these moods and this apathy, but it's the hardest thing in the world. If I go out, all I can think about is getting home and away from people. I who used to stand on a stage night after night, completely composed."

TRUCULENCE AND IRRITABILITY

Women who have always been charming and easy going, suddenly get truculent, difficult, intolerant and downright bitchy with people, and know that they are acting out of character, but cannot help it. They get screaming mad at others for small misdemeanours, and can tear their families to shreds by this behaviour.

"I have turned, so I am told, from a charming gay witty person into a sour embittered cantankerous woman, who is jealous of everyone with a car and a man. I was never like this before. I can only think that the 'change' has completely changed my personality."

The tragedy here lies in the words 'so I am told', for who could have told her this? A member of her family, or a friend, or just an acquaintance. Whoever did was either ignorant of her menopausal condition or deliberately trying to hurt her and make things worse, or even perhaps at the end of their own tether because she was continually being difficult. This quote pathetically reveals the enormous need for sympathy and understanding from others which women who do suffer difficult emotional problems need; a sympathy which it may, for others, be all too hard to give and especially to keep on giving.

APATHY

Some women feel that they just can't be bothered any longer with running their homes or even looking after themselves.

"I could look at dust and dirt around the home and

ignore it for weeks. I did not bath or change my clothes for weeks, whereas previously I had been a daily bather and changed at least once a day."

This kind of behaviour could be a revolt against having spent a long time being a good housewife, and also a feeling, that 'well, I am getting old and unattractive anyway so why bother'. The psychological motivations of such behaviour cannot be explained in a few words here. What we are concerned with is how to cope with such feelings. This woman had the sense to see her own problems in a detached way, and although she doesn't think she *"has been very good at facing up to menopause"*, she has in fact taken positive action. She *"engaged someone to help with the housework one morning a week so that at least a modicum of family comfort is certain,"* took her daily rest and *"read whatever books I could on the subject."* In this case medical examination found no organic trouble, neither did her doctor bother to suggest to her that her age and menopause could be the problem, nor was any treatment prescribed.

INADEQUACY AND DEPRESSION

So many women feel that for one reason or another, they are inadequate, no longer able to run their homes and look after their families properly. One person's attitude to this problem is very clear from the following quote. *"My biggest problem is lack of self confidence and feelings of inadequacy, and inability to cope, which overwhelm me at times. It helps to know that these will pass, and I am beginning to find out little 'tricks' that help. Concentrating on positive thinking and trying to avoid over-involvement in worries. I find things like gardening, walking and washing clothes calming to the mind when under stress."*

Another woman, highly intelligent and involved in a career as well as family life puts her feelings and attitudes in this way. *"My way is to use depressions. In those moods the cruelty of life becomes clear, not only its ridiculous brevity, but the appalling things human beings do to each other and themselves, and the uselessness of achievement and the tragedy of old age. One can hardly bear to read the newspapers—the nightmareish lack of connection between what humanity wants (or thinks it wants) and what nations and systems do, is so evident that one understands those poor nuts who set fire to themselves in public places. None of this is the result of an individual's depression; the individual has simply been deprived for a while of his or her defences against being sharply aware of it all. It seems to me right that one should at times face it, and I have tried, during those times when I was shoved up against it by physical goings-on in my body, to contemplate it as thoroughly as I can for my soul's good, so to speak. Since I have never gone so far into gloom as to lose sight of its physical cause, or to be unable to foresee its end in a few days time, this hasn't been too testing."*

This is a wonderful example of self-knowledge, but it shows up by contrast the problems of women who suffer enormous depressions, inadequacies and anxieties without understanding them or knowing how to cope with them.

"It is the mental depression and physical tiredness that are such burdens, and when, as in my case, there seems to be no end to the condition, it is indeed a severe trial." The key words here being 'in my case there seems to be no end'. This woman is definitely NOT coping.

"I soon felt so unbalanced and so unsure of myself that I became desperate. The world became a terrifying place to live in. I am unable to visualise a future happy life." Another one who cannot see the way through, and who will suffer much more until menopause passes, as it most certainly will.

THOUGHTS OF DEATH

"I found I could think of nothing else but death and sickness—I was obsessed with them."

"Conviction of being a useless person who would never be able to cope with life and who never had coped, and with a recognisably unreasonable temptation to suicide." Recognisably unreasonable, so in this case probably unlikely ever to happen.

These depressions can reach such a pitch that suicidal thoughts and thoughts of death loom up and in an effort to shake them off, some women uselessly resort to alcohol, or sink into an extremely disturbed state. Stressing yet once again that these feelings and problems are only too real for the sufferer; there is only one answer and that is to seek sympathetic medical help, and to do one's damndest to believe that the symptoms will pass, because they are largely glandular in origin, and for those close to her to be infinitely long suffering and equally knowledgeable and sure of the better days to come, and for the woman herself to be as positive as she can bear to be.

HOW TO COPE WITH MENTAL PROBLEMS

Keep active, find things to do, hobbies or work, and mix with people in whatever circumstances you can. All kinds of women's associations, from women's institutes, to ladies bridge clubs, to various social and welfare organisations devoted to helping others, to lunch clubs, are if one thinks of it, full of women in middle age, many of whom find that these things do take them out of themselves and help enormously. It is perhaps much harder for the working woman, or those who have heavy family responsibilities, for the less well off, to mix with other people in this way, and there is a very big problem here. *"At this time of life you need extra money to go out and buy nice clothes and things, and this helps enormously.*

"This is the time of life when I could use a little extra money. I should spend it on visits to the hairdresser for hair tinting, and private dentistry to fill the gaps, great morale boosters. High protein, low sugar diets are expensive—clothes for the over-weight are also more expensive. However as I have two daughters on grants, plus two younger children, this is the time when money seems to be at its tightest, and I think this makes life very difficult."

What of the women who have no money at all to spare, and whose families are largely unsympathetic through ignorance, and just sweep it all under the carpet as an inescapable part of a woman's existence? Such women and families are unlikely to read this book, or to go to their doctors for help, and these women form an enormous social problem whose edges are barely touched. Even in these days of social concern it is still extremely difficult to get at this particular problem. And one cannot help feeling that many of the difficulties we face with the young, and do try to do something about, might be alleviated a little if the difficulties of their menopausal mothers got more attention, especially as the youngsters' own reactions in later life when they themselves reach menopause, or when their wives do, can be very much conditioned by what happened to mother all those years ago.

"My first contact with menopause came in the form of fear. I was terrified by my mother's behaviour during what must have been for her an intensely difficult time. I did not know why she hung out of windows, rushed away from the table screaming, etc. Childish misbehaviour seemed to trigger off dramatic scenes and I was a silent petrified child." This woman intelligently decided that when the time came she would remain calm and not let such things happen. Nevertheless, she did have severe problems. Perhaps she had inherited her mother's glandular set up to some extent, perhaps, subconsciously she was still strongly influenced by her memories. But she says she IS making her way through.

LIVING A FULL LIFE DURING AND AFTER MENO-PAUSE

Now to look on the brighter side. Many women feel an upsurge of creative energy, almost amounting to second adolescence. *"I became very much aware of beauty in form and line and colour and produced some quite good poetry."* There is a tremendous sense of relief from the physical problems of being a woman. Many launch off into new careers or take up old skills and burst back into useful life.

"I am undergoing a second adolescence with similar mental characteristics, and I hope that I shall come out of it with a more stable and balanced personality." Another says she took up writing more successfully when she was fifty and a profile of her lists three books, many pamphlets and articles and a whole series of high level committee appointments. She has travelled all over the world for various organisations, and is a woman who while working extremely hard and doing a great deal of important work, has a family and enjoys a perfectly normal life, and has incidentally, only suffered minor menopausal upsets. Maybe she has been lucky in that her glands have treated her well, or maybe it is her drive and activity which have kept her going, probably a bit of both. But it is too easy to say just that she is lucky, and also very irritating to the less happy to hold her up as an example. Suffice to say that change of life isn't always gloom and despair.

There are so many things to do, first of all for those lucky enough to have families, and perhaps grandchildren.

They can take a full, active and responsible part in family life. *"I feel I shall be different and I hope a deeper person than I was in my thirties. More understanding of life. Having experienced difficulties makes one more tolerent of other people."* Because of this older women are often excellent at social work, from full time jobs such as marriage guidance counselling, (which requires training of course) to teaching. They have a mature understanding of human problems. One woman, already a teacher, whose husband died and children left home *"started studying for a higher degree, this led almost at once to an academic job which I thoroughly enjoy."* Others resume or begin a new career. Look round and one sees many middle aged women in high powered jobs in journalism, fashion, the theatre and business. It is a matter of not feeling that one is finished at fifty and of 'taking the plunge' into a new life.

One woman, herself experiencing change of life, has become manageress of an employment agency. She describes some of the problems of menopausal women who are trying to get work. *"A great many of them are going through various stages (of menopause). Those I try to negotiate for who are really unfit for the kind of work they hope to get, humble me enormously in their dogged belief that they can do what I would never try to do. And again there are too many employers who say 'not over 45'. I get this feeling of wanting to protect them, still able and competent, and yet at the same time I am aware of their shortcomings. It is too simple to say that a woman at this age has more to contribute, and too often this is not really the case. Unless she uses her experience to broaden and strengthen her tolerance and insight, she is obviously less useful and certainly less attractive to look at. But I am equally strengthened by someone who gracefully emerges and impresses me with her warmth and humour and courage, and then smiling informs me she is 62. Quality is indeed ageless, and however glorious the surging thrust of youthful discovery, it can never outshine the quiet confidence of having come through and made it."*

Unpaid social work, 'meals on wheels' working as a 'Samaritan', working for Oxfam, etc, can fill up spare time for women who are already quite busy with family responsibilities.

There are voluntary or sometimes part time jobs as secretaries of clubs for young people, etc. We know of a middle aged woman who is the highly successful secretary of a big sailing club. She takes all the organisational work off the shoulders of the young people who just want to be out in their boats, and so is a vital member of a group of people with like interest, of all ages.

And how about this. *"I am indebted to my doctor for the philosophy which sums up my personal findings to date. i.e. immerse yourself in something that interests you and endeavour to set on one side physical and mental inconveniences."*

"I am 53, the mother of three plus an adopted child, plus elderly parents to care for. After a year spent spasmodically in an enduring variety of indefinite complaints which convinced me that life was at an end. This

began with freelance writing, nursing, social work, art school, etc, and came to a head when at 49 I was accepted at a College of Education for a three year course to be a teacher. I was by far the oldest inhabitant and was often taught by someone young enough to be my child. I had to do the well-nigh (for me) impossible in the way of P.E., Dance and Movement, Swimming, not to mention coping with sociology, psychology, philosophy, etc, plus all manner of novelties like pottery, sculpture and oil painting, and dramatics and music. And making my debut in the classrooms under the amused glances of young and terrifying competent teachers. All this while coping with teenage problems at home, mending socks and peeling potatoes. I have now been teaching for eight months and feel it has been a life saver.''

That long quote sums it all up. From somewhere she has gained the mental and physical energy literally to take up her bed and walk, and really her statement speaks happily and entirely for itself.

4 Sexual Problems

Marital Relationships .. Risk of Conception .. The Contraceptive Pill .. Hysterectomy .. Vaginal Shrinkage .. Climacteric or Change of Life in Men .. Perverted Sexual Feelings.

MARITAL RELATIONSHIPS

In the old days women were brought up to believe that they were not meant to enjoy sexual intercourse. Sex was, as far as they were concerned, only a means to an end:—the production of children. That any decent woman should actually enjoy sex, and especially should continue to enjoy it during and after menopause, was a shocking thought. Thank heavens these ideas are a thing of the past. Yet there is still a vague memory of them around, because we women now in change of life, had mothers who, if they got any sex education or guidance at all, learnt these archaic ideas. Our mothers were young women during the twenties and early thirties, a time of great liberation for women, and most of them discarded these ideas. Nevertheless, some of them did rub off a little onto us, and onto their sons, our husbands.

This is one reason why many middle aged couples find it hard to talk between themselves about their sexual problems, and why both sexes still have some strange preconceived ideas about sex during menopause.

First a fact:—The physical capacity for sexual enjoyment does not alter at all because of change of life. Whether or not a woman wants more or less sex during change is largely emotional and will be discussed below. But it cannot be stressed too strongly that nothing whatsoever happens to her physically which makes it any harder to experience orgasm, and to enjoy sex just as much as she always had. In fact many women can and do until real old age just makes them too tired to bother!

Most women who have had reasonably happy married lives and have borne children, greet menopause hopefully as a time which may bring its immediate small problems, but will mean the end of a lot of worry about possible pregnancy, and a chance to 'let go' and enjoy their sex lives as never before because childbearing is past.

"Far from having problems, I feel nothing but thankfulness for being free from all that boring mess, and joyous anticipation of a sex life without precautions."

This also applies to some single women. *"If I am safely over the boring business of menopause, then I will certainly behave in a free and easy manner."*

Those for whom sex was only a means to the end of producing children, may have a completely opposite reaction, and once their excuse for sex has gone, feel a total revulsion against it.

Single women, widows who don't feel they have had enough children, or childless married women, sometimes go through hell because they realise that now they cannot have children; and the sexual urges which they have for years channelled off into something else; teaching, creative work, or a career, or into short term affairs, increase and worry them. They may have sex dreams, which is a perfectly natural way for the mind and body to get rid, quite harmlessly, of excess sexual feelings. But to some women sex dreams are very upsetting and they are badly shocked by their own dreams. They feel intense shame, thereby exaggerating other worry and anxiety symptoms from which they may be suffering as a result of glandular imbalance. Women obviously find it hard to talk to their doctors or even to their friends about these dreams, and to these one can only stress that these dreams are just a natural safety valve for sexual feelings which cannot be expressed in any other way, and they are absolutely nothing to be ashamed of, whatever form they take.

For various reasons, not entirely understood, many women undoubtedly do feel increased sexual desires and urges during menopause, and if they can be expressed in their relationships with their husbands, they will probably find it a lot easier to get through any other difficulties— hot flushes, etc, because there will be a continuance of married happiness and a closeness to their men which will make things easier all round.

A man whose wife experienced vastly increased sexual urges, which he did not realise, finally discovered by chance that she was indulging her sexual desires with other men, and in a highly intense and sometimes abnormal way.

He was horrified, but loved his wife, and after initial rows, had the sense to try to put things to rights. He came to the conclusion that he quite simply hadn't been an exciting enough lover for her, and that he would try to be in the future. This worked, and both of them have settled down to a new and obviously much more satisfactory sex life. The past is not referred to and with luck they will live to a ripe and happy old age! *"In our particular case much more patience, tenderness and physical contact should have been shown by me at the onset of my wife's menopause. A husband should build up constant nearness and feelings of physical oneness and cherishing love—as was openly demonstrated in the days of courtship before marriage. Another thing is to discuss openly and without laughing derisively exactly what the wife wants and feels at the time of menopause. Shyness must be overcome, and tenderness and sympathy always shown; however odd may be the effects of menopause from the purely male observer's point of view!"*

"What I can't understand is why sexual feelings keep on developing at this late stage of ones life, until one is really afraid of any close contact, yet ten years before I had become incapable of the sex act." This woman who has suffered a very difficult menopause mentally is obviously very disturbed by her rejection of physical sex, which is built up into emotional sex, and physical feelings which are not finding expression.

It is much harder for women who, as noted above, feel a partial or total revulsion against sex. Maybe they only associate sex with having children, maybe they feel that they and their husbands are getting old and the whole thing is a bit ridiculous. Or that their husbands are bored with being tied to an ageing woman *"who feels somewhat on the scrap heap, because she has reached menopause."*

Other women report as follows:—

"A distinct falling off of sexual energy in the last year. I still like to make love for emotional reasons but feel that at times as though the emotions were linked to the genitals by one particular nerve and that nerve had been cut. I have to play-act a bit."

Maybe they have never been particularly keen and feel that this is the chance to drop the whole thing, using change of life as an excuse. Some women feel revulsion to their husbands but at the same time are attracted to other men. *"as far as I can sort out my own menopause problems, it seems to have begun when I became infatuated with a man I really didn't like at all. My marriage was a very strong one, and didn't break, but I certainly felt resentment towards my husband without any reason, because he was a truly loving and gentle man. When my husband made love to me I just could not prevent the tears flowing, such was the strength of this infatuation."*

"As for resuming the sexual side of one's life—it is something I dread. I feel just nothing inside, only a dread when my husband makes an approach to me, and before, I was an extremely warm and passionate woman."

"My married life is negligible. From being a normal

woman with a happy sex life, I now have no feelings whatsoever. My husband is kind and understanding and realises how I feel so it is now a thing of the past. I mentioned this to a specialist and asked if my feelings would revert to normal, and he said 'Possibly, possibly not'. So that is that. I feel I could scream if my husband came anywhere near me, yet I idolise him." This is an extreme reaction, and the specialist's remark pinpoints yet again the impossibility of giving pat answers in such cases.

There are so many complex emotional reasons for such feelings. For women whose husbands are understanding, an escape to separate bedrooms, and mutual release from sexual demands at least for the time being may be the answer, and other anxieties will lessen in proportion. But for a woman whose husband cannot or will not understand, who finds it very difficult indeed to make do with less sex, or no sex, things can become very difficult. She may manage by just being passive, but being a passive sexual partner can lead to a desperate feeling of resentment against what she comes to feel are selfish sexual demands. Although she may fully realise that by depriving her husband of his sexual outlet, she is upsetting him dreadfully, bewildering him, and possibly driving him to other women. If she loves him deeply she will suffer much guilt from her own behaviour yet know she cannot alter it without being 'used', and resentments build up both ways between husbands and wives.

Many husbands just cannot understand why wives with whom they have always been happy lovers, suddenly seem to find them repulsive. They in turn get anxious, take an extra drink or two, or get resentful. All these states take an awful lot of sympathy, understanding and unselfishness on both sides. *"My husband has been most wonderfully kind and helpful, but I have been so dismal I would not have blamed him if he had lost interest in me."*

When menopause is passing many women revert to the sexual attitudes they felt before it ever started; but meanwhile separate bedrooms, rows, misunderstandings, guilt, other women, other men, grey hairs, etc, have intervened, and it can be extremely difficult to find the way back to life together and relationships as they were before. It is awfully hard for men to know when they can be 'reinstated', as it were, or for women to make it clear to them that things can go back to normal. This is why husbands and wives who love each other, or who are happy together and don't wish to break up a perfectly good marriage or to spend the rest of their lives either bickering or in withdrawn silence, should try hard, during menopause, to talk about it as much as possible, or if they just can't do that, to keep as close together as they can in every other way, so that if and when things return to their own particular normal, they can do so easily. There is always the 'if'. Many couples work out a way of living together without much or any physical sex, and are content that things should remain this way as they go through middle and old age.

One can only stress again that all these problems are so invidual and so varied that no sweeping comprehensive advice is possible. For some couples the marriage guidance counsellor may be a great help, and those who feel that they can talk to one, either singly or together, should try this source of help.

RISK OF CONCEPTION

The danger of unwanted conception is no greater than at any other time, provided contraceptive precautions are kept up as they have been throughout life, until at least one year, and for complete safety, two years, after the final period. For those whose contraceptive methods have always been a bit haphazard, then intercourse followed by about two or three months without a period can be very worrying indeed, because you just don't know whether you are pregnant or simply irregular. There are two courses of action. First, get some sound advice on contraception from your doctor or a family planning clinic. Secondly, if you do miss a period and are not certain, don't spend two or three months worrying, go straight to your doctor and get a pregnancy test done. At least your mind will be at rest one way or the other.

THE CONTRACEPTIVE PILL AND MENOPAUSE

The pros and cons of the use of the 'Pill' are not in the scope of this book. Various versions of the oral pill have been produced, but they all work by regulating the ovulatory and menstrual cycle by administering regular doses of hormones. Now that the pill has been in widespread use for some years it is known that while many women feel no ill effects from them whatsoever, and some medical conditions are benefited positively by taking the hormones, there are women who develop conditions attributable to the extra supplies of hormones. In particular, doctors are advised by the makers of the pills and by those who have researched it, that women over the age of 35 are more likely to suffer ill effects than younger women. If it is prescribed for older women they should be checked regularly for ill effects. Yet there is a school of thought which believes that a woman who takes the pill regularly for years will not suffer menopause symptoms to such a degree as she would had she not taken it.

However, as older women are not usually advised to use the pill, most of those now approaching, experiencing, or passing out of change of life will NOT have been taking the pill. If they have done so, their doctors must have prescribed it and therefore should be prepared to cope with any problems which may occur.

There are widely conflicting schools of thought in the medical profession about the effects of the pill generally and on menopausal women in particular. Until more time has passed and more research been done, as the younger women who have been taking the pill for years, reach menopause, no hard and fast conclusions can be drawn.

Sone young women on the pill suffer depression, nausea, pigmentation, obesity, headaches and other symptoms often associated with menopause, and the conclusion must be that these are caused by hormone imbalance arising from taking the pill. This should make it even more clear to those who believe that change of life symptoms are 'all in the mind' that they are wrong and that these things are sparked off by hormone imbalance.

HYSTERECTOMY

Hysterectomy is the surgical operation which removes the womb. Total hysterectomy with bi-lateral ovarectomy removes the womb and both ovaries. This may become necessary to clear up gynaecological troubles not in the scope of this book. Suffice it to say that if the operation is recommended by your doctors, while it is no laughing matter, it is a 'good' operation and is highly successful in its results. The removal of the womb does not affect other organs, nor does it affect physical sexual enjoyment, except it obviously means no more children. For many it means getting rid of a load of trouble and a new feeling of security and freedom from worry. If the womb is removed before menopause, and one or both ovaries are left behind, menopause will take place in due course as it would have done anyway (although of course periods will have ceased with the removal of the womb), but there will be no anxieties about irregular periods, risk of cancer, or pregnancy, etc. Other menopausal symptoms, due to the slowing down of the oestrogen supply from the ovaries, will occur in relation to the efficiency with which your endocrine system compensates. A woman may have hot flushes, anxieties, depressions, or sail through the whole thing with serenity, because she is not anxious.

But if the hysterectomy has been total and both ovaries

have gone, then within a short while, whatever the age of the woman, menopausal symptoms may occur because the oestrogen supply has been suddenly stopped. *"After my operation I went through a short, sharp menopause."*

"An extended total hysterectomy projected me at the stroke of knives into the state at 35 years of age."

Doctors know this may happen, and it would seem to be their responsibility to make this clear to the patient beforehand; and after the operation, to take steps to balance out the hormones medically. Undoubtedly many doctors do this, but some do not. The patients of these doctors are taken by surprise when they start menopausal symptoms. *"Prior to having my hysterectomy I had read a booklet which said that any woman undergoing this was always most carefully looked after by her doctor—that was where the joke was on me. I left hospital, not even being told to see my doctor, or what to expect."* This woman has a great many symptoms and complains that even for the physical ones such as irritation of the vagina *"Nothing has been done."* This is perhaps an extreme case, and it would be quite wrong to suggest that all doctors behave this way; but cases do occur, and cannot be brushed aside. One can only stress that all women faced by a total hysterectomy should ask their doctors about what menopausal symptoms they may expect, and make sure that if they do experience any, they keep asking for help. Remember always that the symptoms are very definitely physical (endocrinal) in origin.

Some doctors feel that to tell a woman before the

operation that she may be projected into menopause, is to give her an added load of worry about the future, at a time when she should be as little worried as possible. This is fair enough, provided that after the operation she is told to refer to her doctor if she experiences menopausal symptoms, which should be described to her. *"Nobody had told me anything regarding potential consequences and how to overcome problems arising there from . . . However, I am an intellectual (they tell me) and solve difficulties first by an academic, theoretical, then by an active practical approach. Knowing this my doctor has lent me all his textbooks on my return from hospital."* She goes on to describe her severe symptons and deep depression, and how she overcame them after a year, and now several years later she feels fine. This is a prime example of an intelligent and sensible woman and an intelligent and sensible doctor sorting out a problem between them. Doctors cannot be expected to lend their textbooks to all their patients, and quite rightly feel strongly that 'a little knowledge is a dangerous thing' in the sense that it can lead to wrong self-diagnosis and wrong self-treatment. The failure is one communication. This book tries to open up the lines of communication. It is isolation with one's worries, from one's doctor and the rest of humanity, which makes them so hard to cope with. *"I need advice on these matters; but somehow or another, I have no-one to discuss things with."*

SHRINKAGE OF THE VAGINA

This condition, known medically as Kraurosis, is not at all common although some women do suffer from it progressively towards the end of menopause, after periods have finished. It takes the form of itching or slight pain at the entrance of the vagina, and sometimes it may become painful to sit or to urinate. There may be unpleasant discomfort or pain during intercourse. *"I have found that occasionally the vaginal secretions seem to be absent, which means discomfort with dryness and tightness; but I have found vaseline to be a great help."*

The condition can be helped enormously by oestrogen ointments or by oestrogen tablets. A non-greasy surgical lubricant which can be bought from any chemist, is very helpful when used before intercourse. Possibly the most difficult aspect of this particular problem is that such measures may be off-putting for the woman who has never had sexual problems, and if she is going through a phase when sex is repugnant to her, this can make it even more so.

CLIMACTERIC OR CHANGE OF LIFE IN MEN

Do men go through some form of change of life? Obviously they don't suffer the big physical and endocrinal changes that affect women, but some men definitely do pass through a kind of change of life. As they begin to age their sexual urges may gradually decrease, and they may suffer a lot of anxiety and depression over what they feel to be loss of virility or potency. So much so that they seek sexual intercourse with their wives infrequently. If their wives are also menopausal this may be quite the wrong thing. Those women whose sexual urges increase during and after change can feel very let down by an undemanding husband, and far from realising that he himself is having problems, think that the fault is theirs and that they are no longer attractive. This can lead to an awful lot of misunderstanding and unhappiness. When a married couple talk together and are not diffident about discussing themselves, they can more easily work things out without resentment. When a pair can't talk together, there may be a build-up leading to all kinds of misunderstandings. A woman may feel that, if her husband isn't interested in her, she has to prove she is still attractive by finding another man. And likewise a man whose sexual powers are on the wane, and whose wife isn't particularly interested in sex, may try to revitalise and prove himself by finding another and perhaps younger woman. We have already quoted the case of the woman who formed some bizarre sexual relationships, which were discovered by her husband. He set about putting things right by stepping up his own performance as a lover and the pair have literally taken on a new lease of life and love.

All human beings possess varying quantities of hormones which produce varying types, from the excessively masculine man, through the more feminine man and the more masculine woman, to the excessively feminine woman. So it is a physiological fact that some men, at middle age, as hormone productions slows and alters, can experience some of the symptoms common to women—hot flushes, obesity, depression, headaches, though not in so marked a way. Many men would reject utterly any suggestion that they may be suffering from a reduction of female hormones in their systems, as being an insult to their masculinity, but those who really try to think about their own and their wives problems can accept such ideas privately without feeling ridiculous. Exactly as with women, the symptoms will pass as the hormone balance reasserts itself.

Some men suffer slight pregnancy sickness and even labour pains, in sympathy with their pregnant wives, and no-one really understands the powerful psychological factors which produce this sympathetic reaction. Some people believe that male changes of life, when it takes place as the same time as that of a much loved wife, is the same kind of thing.

PERVERTED SEXUAL URGES

What does or does not constitute perversion is really a matter for the individual to decide. In the terms of this book and for each individual woman, perhaps the best definition is that she finds herself wishing for sexual relationships or sexual acts which she has not consciously sought before, and which by a lifetime of conditioning and social habit seem to her to be perverted. Sexual acts between men and women can take very simple or very complicated forms. To the person whose sex life has been simple. The complicated forms may seem to be perversions, which strictly speaking they are not. Homosexual feelings and desires may horrify some women, yet to others seem to be more natural than heterosexual feelings. Sex dreams, masturbation and self-stimulation are common and not to be considered unnatural, especially in women living alone. The fact that in many women different and exaggerated sexual desires may appear and be gratified when they have always been repressed, during change of life, is hard to explain briefly. It is a very complex psychological problem. Possibly the sense of release from responsibilities towards one's family, freedom from fears of more childbearing, and a determination to enjoy the rest of active life, that one has previously suppressed, triggers off indulgence in sexual experimentation.

Women for whom heterosexual relationships have been unsatisfactory or non-existent, may, when they suddenly realise that life is passing them by, decide to throw convention to the winds and take their sex where they want it. Lesbian relationships are often formed when one or other partner is passing through change of life.

Undoubtedly anything which a woman herself feels to be perverted and 'wrong' will cause her to feel guilty, which can lead to or exaggerate other menopausal anxieties. The woman who finds that she is gaining sexual release and happiness from 'perverted' sex, should accept this state of affairs without guilt, without anxiety, provided that she is not damaging other people. She should accept that her sexuality, though its object and its expression may be, in the eyes of society, perverted, is finding what is for her, a normal outlet, which will help her through the other difficulties of change of life.

The woman who is totally unable to accept her own 'perverted' desires without guilt, may be helped by a psychologist to understand, control, and perhaps to pass through these feelings without carrying quite such a weight of guilt as she feels alone.

Menopausal women often find themselves sexually attracted to men and boys, donkey's years younger than themselves, and this can be very strong. Their own adolescent children's friends may attract them. Usually women form a kind of mother relationship with their children's friends which channels off some of this feeling, but it can be extremely intense and sometimes reciprocated, temporarily at any rate. This leads into very deep waters indeed, every woman knows this, but it causes extra strain by its necessary repression. But she must realise that such feelings are neither abnormal nor perverted; no cause for guilt, just for commonsense.

TREATMENT

Any woman who feels that she is really in a state because of sexual problems, dreams, desires, etc., and just cannot cope, should seek the help of a psychiatrist. It may not be possible for you to talk about such intimate matters to your family doctor, but if you can bring yourself to tell him at least that you have sexual problems which you would like to discuss with a psychiatrist, he should put you into touch with one.

CONCLUSIONS

Change of life is a time through which all women must pass, now that we are no longer worn out by continual childbearing and do live to a ripe old age. Its problems will, ninety-nine times out of a hundred, disappear as the hormone systems of the body adjust themselves. Yet the problems can be severe and are very real. They are not all in the mind but are physical in origin. Yet such is the power of mind over body that they can be made worse or better according to the attitudes of the sufferer. Lucky the woman who is so controlled that she can push her problems under the carpet and sail through it all, and lucky too the woman whose body adjusts itself so well that her problems are slight anyway. Unlucky the woman who has many problems and finds herself overwhelmed by them.

It helps so much to talk to someone who is medically trained or trained in social work, or to a wise friend, especially to an older woman who is well and truly back in circulation again.

There are medical treatments which may help a lot, but there is still much research to be done, so don't blame your doctor if he cannot provide an immediate answer out of a bottle of pills.

Your family must realise that mother is going through a trying time, and teenage children should not present her with great piles of dirty clothes, untidy rooms, and demand enormous meals all the time. They, and husbands, however helpless they have been in the past, just cannot expect the same or more work from mother on chores and housework. Families MUST realise this and buckle to and help. No one is suggesting that they overdo this to the point where mother can sit around all day with her feet up, this is self defeating, for it is essential that a woman keeps as busy as she can manage without fatigue.

Change of life, menopause, call it what you will, is not a killer. We should be very badly off for grandmothers if it were. We older women are an enormously important section of our society, and do so much work in hundreds of ways that society would be hard put to it to do without us.

Keep these things in mind when menopause and its difficulties and depressions have brought you low, and look forward to a lot of the best of life which is still to come. You are not alone, you are not unique, you can be helped, and you can help yourself.

ABOUT THE AUTHOR.

Suzanne Beedell, is aged 50, is married (her husband is aged 51). She has two daughters, one aged 23 is married. The second is aged 8.

Suzanne Beedell has written books and articles on many subjects. This book is an objective discussion of a subject in which she feels herself to be deeply involved, and has been written to clear up misconceptions and to put forward positive ideas, and to open up a human problem which has been, in the past, bypassed and swept under the carpet.